The Dangers of Denial

Lonseth

Embracing the Challenges of Alzheimers and Dementia

By

ELIZABETH LONSETH

ISBN: 1512069019
ISBN: 9781512069013

Dedication and Thanks

To my parents and in-laws who struggled with memory disease.

A special thanks to my husband, Stan Lonseth, for his continued support and cover photography. "After The Storm" is the perfect cover photo.

With gratitude to Nancy Nelson for her support in writing this booklet.

Thank you to my friend, Carol Lee Clayton, for again working together and sharing the journey.

A portion of the proceeds from the sale of this booklet will be donated to the Alzheimer's Association.

To find out more about Elizabeth Lonseth and her other publications, please visit www.elizabethlonsethnovels.com

To see additional photography by Stan Lonseth, please visit www.capobeachphotography.com

Foreword

Jeffery Anderson, feature writer for A Place for Mom:

In *The Dangers of Denial,* Elizabeth Lonseth's straight talk about dementia caregiving will help families to see the reality of their situation and their loved one's condition, while at the same time providing them the tools and information they need to cope.

Lonseth has a powerful, compassionate, and informal voice that easily connects with fellow caregivers. Her experience helping to care for her in-laws and her own parents during their autumn years has provided her a wealth of knowledge from which to draw, and her caregiving parables are a testament to the teaching power of the narrative form.

Lonseth demonstrates skill crystallizing broad and difficult topics to their core, conveying essential information while simultaneously respecting the scarce time of the caregivers who are her readers.

I would recommend *The Dangers of Denial* to any dementia caregiver.

Maria Connelly, National Wellness Team Leader, Kisco Senior Living:

I found this book a valuable resource that focuses specifically on facing the denial of Alzheimer's "head-on". The emotional and physical toll on families, caregivers, and friends is well addressed in this book. I believe *The Dangers of Denial* is an invaluable guide in helping with these issues.

The book provides an easy to understand, concise, and pro-active approach when dealing with the denial that everyone experiences. It also shares many heartfelt and relatable stories that help in understanding what others have experienced.

This is a must read for all who are facing the Alzheimer's journey.

Keri Pollock, Assistant Director of Strategic Initiatives, Office of the Dean, University of Washington School of Nursing, former Marketing Director for the Alzheimer's Association Western and Central Washington Chapter:

"Knowledge is power," and after caring for her parents and in-laws, Elizabeth has knowledge to share and life experience from which readers can greatly benefit. Let her knowledge be your power. Don't deny (pun intended) yourself a quick read which will help you start down the path of understanding and acceptance. This book is the perfect place to start.

Preface

I am not a doctor, a scientist or a specialist. I am simply a person who has taken the journey of being a caregiver to a dementia patient four times. My parents and my in-laws experienced some form of memory disease.

In the late 1980s, following fourteen years of heart attacks and strokes, my father began suffering from vascular dementia. In my mid-thirties — with a husband, three daughters, and a career in interior design — I was in full denial. My father was still in the beginning stages of dementia when he passed away from a heart attack in 1990.

Seven years later we began the long eight-year journey with my in-laws. At first we checked on them several times a day, making sure they were still fixing their meals, paying the bills, and not burning the house down. Within a few years this routine snowballed on us, and for another six years we were providing full-time care. Without any prior planning it sucked us in and it seemed there was no way out. My father-in-law had Alzheimer's and my mother-in-law had vascular dementia. We took turns caring for them; bathing, toileting, and feeding them. Our three daughters helped out at various times, and we hired occasional in-home help.

My in-laws passed away four months apart, in 2005. Just a few months later my mother started showing signs of Alzheimer's. My first reaction was anger. I did not want to go down that road again. For several months I wrestled with the reality of my mom's condition. Then armed with the knowledge and experience I had gained over the previous eight years, and with a larger budget, I faced the disease head on — or so I thought.

For several years I organized in-home care for Mom. During that time my husband and I had purchased a new home. Due to our work we were spending part of each week in California and part of each week living on our boat in Seattle. As Mom became less mobile and needed assistance in the bathroom, we had to move her to a memory care facility. Her home was a split-level design with steep stairs. The bathrooms Mom had designed were so small they would make airplane designers jealous. Now my mother is in the later stages of Alzheimer's and is receiving excellent care in a facility close to my home in California. I have finally learned to embrace the reality of the disease.

In the past two years I have had the honor of speaking at senior living facilities throughout the United States. Before and after each presentation I try to talk to family members in attendance, hoping to learn from their experiences. Often the stories I hear break my heart, but I keep listening, yearning for new tips or examples that might help someone else traveling this long, lonely journey.

Table of Contents

Note:
This booklet has been developed from public talks given on the subject of denial and is written in a more conversational style than my earlier booklet, *A Gradual Disappearance.*

The information available about memory disease is being updated constantly as new tests and research projects yield new conclusions. I have tried to provide current and correct information available at the time of publication.

Introduction

One of the biggest obstacles in getting proper care for memory patients is denial. As human beings we often avoid problems or hurtful situations to protect our emotions. By denying that problems exist, we hope to avoid mental or emotional pain.

When starting to write about denial in regard to dementia, I decided to do some research on the earth's largest bird, thinking it would be a great example. I checked zoo websites — did you know that ostriches don't really put their heads in the sand to hide from their problems? It was the Roman writer Pliny the Elder who, in his *Naturalis Historia* gave the ostrich a bad reputation. Apparently, Pliny didn't get close enough to really check things out.

There are three behaviors ostriches demonstrate that give the illusion they are putting their heads in the sand. First of all, they bury their large eggs in the sand, and with their beaks they turn them every so often. So that does involve sticking their beaks in the sand, not to avoid problems, but to care for their young. Second, they eat small pebbles and gravel to help digest their food. While they collect the gravel, they keep their heads close to the ground. Third, when they sense danger, their first instinct is to run, but at times they elect to stay put and become part of the scenery. With their heads down on the ground, not in it, their plumage sticks up and it blends well with the surrounding shrubbery. Sometimes they put their heads next to the ground and kneel down. Their head and neck blend in with the sand and dirt, and their bodies look like just another bush in the desert.

The ostrich is not trying to avoid its problems; it is caring, resourceful, and assesses each danger, choosing which defense mechanism to use. It is we humans who like to stick our heads in the sand and are selective about which reality we will accept.

Chapter 1

Embracing the Reality of the Disease

"Refusal to admit the truth or reality" is the second definition of "denial" in the free Merriam-Webster Dictionary. As a mechanism we use to protect ourselves from facing a hurtful truth, denial can surface in many areas of our lives. It can make us feel temporarily better. It can be a good tool when we need a little time or space to adjust to a new or a shocking situation. However, remaining in a state of denial will result in additional problems caused by our failure to face reality. This is especially true when dealing with Alzheimer's or dementia.

When discussing denial and memory disease we need to answer the question of who is in the denial: is it the patient, those around the patient, or both?

In the early stages of memory disease patients can be very aware that their minds are slipping away or that their thought processes are changing. Concern might prompt them to initiate the first doctor's appointment. If the disease is diagnosed early enough, family members might have the privilege of creating a care plan with their loved one's participation. I have met a few people in the early stages who have walked up to me and said, "Hi, I am Sally, and I am in the early stages of Alzheimer's." The first few times that happened I paused and didn't quite know what to say. It is unusual that memory patients fully comprehend and openly admit to their disease.

Recently I have had the privilege of getting to know poet Nancy Nelson, who is in the beginning stages of Alzheimer's. She has written a book of poetry on her experiences and calls her Alzheimer's the As to go along with her upbeat positive outlook on life. Nancy is traveling and enjoying life, determined not to let the diagnosis get the better of her. Her family has accepted the diagnosis and is discussing the future with their mother. They have been researching Alzheimer's with her and understand her wishes and concerns. It is a full team effort. Early diagnosis can be a blessing as it allows for more proactive involvement and planning between patients and their loved ones or caregivers.

People may be scared when they first experience memory lapses and try to hide them. It takes energy to focus enough to seem normal in front of others. They might succeed for an hour or so, saying the right things at the right time or not repeating the same question over and over. But as their energy drains, their confusion becomes evident. Memory patients often use humor as a coping mechanism. It makes them feel better, especially when someone laughs at their jokes. They can rationalize, "I'm not so bad off if I can still make people laugh." By using humor, putting on a good front, and limiting their visiting time with others, they can slip through the cracks and avoid early diagnosis.

Family members and friends may not recognize signs of dementia in the early stage concerning their loved ones, such as odd behavior, repetition, or forgetfulness. When memory patients reach the midlevel or advanced stage, they are seldom able to understand or comprehend that they have Alzheimer's or dementia. Family members or caregivers have to be the ones to face the facts. At this point in time scientists have not yet found a cure, so patients are not going to get better — they will only deteriorate. Consequently, family members are left making major decisions (legal and otherwise) as the patient declines. Objectivity becomes necessary not only for the family but also for faithful friends and caring attendants to ensure that the patient receives the best possible care. Unfortunately, a diagnosis is usually determined in the middle or advanced stage of dementia or Alzheimer's.

I received an email from a brother-sister team who were totally overwhelmed with trying to care for both of their parents with Alzheimer's. The sister lived in another state and was worn out from traveling to help out. Their first of many questions was, "How do we get our parents to accept the fact they have Alzheimer's? We remind them several times each day. They keep acting out and we can't keep going on this way." I explained that their parents didn't have to accept the diagnosis, and the constant reminders throughout the day were antagonizing them. They dropped the subject, got rid of some other agitation factors and brought in help. Things are going more smoothly now.

There are different levels of denial in friends and family members. The first level is not accepting that a loved one has the disease. This can be a confusing time not only for the patient, but for the family members too. There are times when a loved one is no longer making sense.

Observers (family members or others) often have these kinds of questions running through their mind: *Why are they acting like this? Why do they keep calling ten times an hour asking the same question over and over? Have they been taking their medications? Why can't they seem to find matching shoes or socks? Are they eating their meals?* We notice the pantry is full of cookies and cakes from the bakery, and the freezer is full of ice cream. *Was it a joke when we overheard them tell a friend that they liked eating dessert for breakfast, lunch, and dinner? But yesterday when they came for dinner, they told jokes, and they remembered all about the 1993 camping trip, every detail.* They have *to be OK.*

We start to help out by bringing them an occasional meal, taking them shopping, and ordering their medication and refills. Somehow running the life of our aging loved ones takes twice as much time as running our own. Between work, the kids or grandkids, and our parents, life is getting out of control. As you talk to friends, they suggest your parents might have dementia. "Oh, no," we say, trying to hide how offended we are. We dismiss it by answering, "They're just a little forgetful. They seem fine most of the time."

Watch out! The train wreck is just about to happen, a train wreck that I have now observed many times with friends and family members.

We need to stop, face the facts, get advice, research, and put a plan in place. Then we will start to bring a sense of order to our lives again. Let's analyze what I just said. Hidden in the questions were hints of memory disease. Loss of communication skills, repetition, and short-term memory loss are all signs. Often the patients can remember every detail from their childhood, young adult years, and even that camping trip twenty-two years ago. But can they remember what they had for dinner last night or the name of their new grand-child? Or that they even have a new grandchild? Don't brush this behavior off as just being a little senile or eccentric. Start investigating the situation more deeply — and sooner rather than later is better.

Some of us will escape memory disease, but as the numbers seem to mushroom we need to be aware of the symptoms. The Alzheimer's Association at (http://www.alz.org/alzheimers_ disease_know_the_10_signs.asp) has a list of ten symptoms to watch for:

1. Memory loss that disrupts daily life
2. Challenges in planning or solving problems
3. Difficulty completing familiar tasks at home, at work, or at leisure
4. Confusion with time or place
5. Trouble understanding visual images and spatial relationships
6. New problems with words in speaking or writing
7. Misplacing things and losing the ability to retrace steps
8. Decreased or poor judgment
9. Withdrawal from work or social activities
10. Changes in mood and personality [1]

Often family members will tell me that their loved one doesn't have Alzheimer's but they just can't remember what day it is, that they no longer want to read or write, and that they are constantly misplacing their wallet or purse. They emphatically start the next sentence with, "They don't have Alzheimer's..." but then continue to describe another symptom from the list. I have met people working in the medical field — for example, a social worker, and a doctor — who were unable to face the fact that *their* parent had memory disease. It is easy to recognize symptoms in other elderly people, but not in your own parent or spouse. The sooner you accept that your loved one or ones have Alzheimer's or dementia the easier your journey will become.

Unlike cancer or heart disease where advances in treatments and medicines have occurred, Alzheimer's doesn't have a cure, a significantly effective medication, or procedures with which to fight the progression of the disease. Therefore, we tend to want to ignore it. However, since 2013, Alzheimer's has officially been the sixth leading cause of death in the United States,[2] and some doctors are predicting it will soon jump to number three.[3] It is now the third leading cause of death in Washington State and North Dakota, and the fifth in California.[4]

We *cannot* ignore it. We have to grow up and face the facts. As the family caregiver or overseer of our loved one's care we need a plan of attack so that the disease does not take us down with it. We need to learn to embrace the reality of the disease.

Chapter 2

Dangers of Denial for the Patient

Refusing to accept that your loved one has Alzheimer's or dementia can lead to bigger problems. Without proper supervision and care, your loved one could get lost, hurt themselves or others, have a home accident, suffer from poor nourishment, cause an accident while driving, overdose on medications, or become a victim of elder abuse.

Getting Lost

Getting lost is a real danger. Occasionally we hear on the local news about an elderly person who is missing and then days later there is another report about finding them alive, or in some sad cases, deceased. They walk away or drive off, not knowing where they are going and cannot find their way home.

Some patients become restless and pace or roam. If they are not supervised they can quickly disappear. During the early stages of his Alzheimer's disease, while recuperating from a surgery, my father-in-law spent a week in a rehabilitation center. We visited often, but on the day of his discharge, we arrived to find an empty room. None of the staff knew where he was. He had wandered out the front door of the facility fully dressed, and because he looked like he knew what he was doing, he had slipped out undetected. After an hour my husband found his father several blocks away in a Safeway store, going up and down the aisles, shopping, but without a wallet.

My father-in-law had been taking the same afternoon walk around his neighborhood every day for years. He continued to do so into the middle-stage of the disease. He would chat with neighbors, checking on the progress of remodeling or landscaping projects. Neighbors would inform us of interesting things he said that didn't add up and we informed them of his situation. One day, while on his daily route, he got lost, and a kind neighbor showed him the way home. As a result of that incident, he became afraid to leave the house, even with one of us accompanying him.

Where my mother currently lives, there was one gentleman who was a "runner," constantly moving and trying to find his way out. His wife had placed him in the senior residence because she could no longer keep him safely at home. The caregivers at the facility could not allow this gentleman out in the beautiful garden by himself, as he could quickly scale the six-foot high ornamental fence and outrun the youngest caregiver. Even with supervised care in a closed environment it may be difficult to keep some patients safe.

Hurting Themselves or Others

Not dealing with increased agitation and restlessness occurring at the end of the day, known as sundown syndrome,[5] could allow the agitation to increase to the point that patients hurt themselves or others. Unfortunately 'acting out' — such as throwing things, hitting, biting, or kicking others — can be a part of the disease. Often patients quickly forget what they have done or attribute their negative actions to someone else, accusing someone else of biting or hitting them. Studies vary but about 20 percent of memory patients become violent.[6] It is important to assess what is triggering the aggression. The unfamiliar setting of a hospital stay, for example, can confuse the patient. Add to that the possibility of adverse medication reactions — say from an antipsychotic or narcotic prescription and even the sweetest little lady could become aggressive.

My mother-in-law required a walker to stabilize her balance, but getting her to use it became impossible. The walker symbolized old age and in her mind she was not old. Due to osteoporosis, she had shrunk more than seven inches and lost over fifty pounds when we introduced the walker to her. We were concerned for her safety because she was so frail. With our encouragement, she would reluctantly use the walker from her bedroom to her living room chair. We would leave it there for her to use and go off to the kitchen or laundry to take care of things. After a few moments we would hear a loud noise. She would gather up every ounce of strength that she had and throw the walker across the living room. We gave up on the walker, as we were afraid she would hurt herself. A physical therapist showed us how to properly use a tightly woven gait belt placed around her waist. With the belt we could walk behind her to provide stability and guide her for short distances in her home.

An article by Dr. Jaya Joy and Dr. Joe John Vattakatucher called "Aggression and violence in patients with dementia," in the April 2013 *GM (Geriatric Medicine) Journal*, describes the need for being objective about your loved one's disease.

Dementia often starts as a problem with cognition but almost always evolves into a problem with behavior. However, no comprehensive guidelines exist on the assessment of risk to others posed by patients with dementia. What constitutes aggression or violence amongst dementia patients is not straightforward. Some nurses would rate behavior as "aggressive" only if the patient intended to harm. The concept of "aggression" and "violence" can be problematic if it depends on "intention to harm" as this may be difficult to assess in this group of patients. [6]

The article goes on to say that with most types of dementia, aggression increases as the severity of the disease increases. However, "fronto-temporal dementia patients are more likely to be aggressive or violent early in the course of disease and they become apathetic and inactive as the disease progresses." [6]

Caregivers need to learn how to approach patients to avoid aggression. Denial will only heighten the problem, as it takes time and training to learn proper methods. If we continually heard the word "No" all day long, I bet by four in the afternoon, or even much earlier, we might also be tempted to act out!

In her article *10 Alternative Ways to Say "No" to Someone With Dementia,* Caring.com contributing editor, Paula Spenser Scott says:

Your goal: to preserve an upbeat, encouraging mood while still managing to set the limits the situation demands. Here are 10 alternatives to "no" that you can try weaving into your vocabulary:

I wish we could!
Wouldn't that be nice?
That's a good idea; let's try to plan something for later.
Would you really like to do that? I didn't know that about you.
I think it's too hot/cold/wet today.
That sounds like fun for next time.
That's an interesting idea to think about.
Oh, I can just imagine that.
*Really? You have so much energy/enthusiasm/imagination/
curiosity.*
I think I'd be more comfortable doing X; sound good? [7]

Using positive responses and vocabulary words that guide will eliminate a lot of agitation. Redirecting their attention to something pleasant when they are agitated with a situation also helps.

Schedule regular doctor appointments as other physical problems can add to a patient's agitation. For example, watch for a urinary tract infection (UTI) or other infections, which can increase confusion and lead to outbursts.

If violence continues to be a problem, it might be time for an appointment with a board certified geriatric psychiatrist. They can assess the situation and determine which of the many medications available can help alleviate the frustration of the patient.

Those of you who remember visiting a nursing home years ago may be hesitant to ask a doctor to prescribe a behavior-modifying medication for your loved one. Aggressive dementia patients back then often sat drooling in their chairs, too doped up to participate in any conversation or activity.

It is very different today. New medications (unavailable to doctors previously) target very specific problems. Geriatric psychiatrists will get to the root cause of the agitation, know which medication to prescribe, and be aware of any side effects. The proper medication if given correctly can make your loved one a happier, and in some cases, a higher functioning person. It will be easier for caregivers to administer proper care, and friends and family will be able to interact with the patient in a positive way.

Accidents in the Home

Accidents in the kitchen can multiply if patients are left unsupervised. As they lose cooking skills, they could cut or burn themselves, leave the stove on, or excessively eat certain foods. Dementia patients are not always aggressive but they forget easily and may not remember how to properly use a knife or scissors.

Fire is a real danger. Unsupervised patients could put a piece of clothing over a lamp to dry. Perhaps they might light candles and forget about them or place them close to a flammable object. They might incorrectly use a space heater, or use the oven for heating the room.

The bathroom presents another set of dangers. The scenario could be getting into the medicine cabinet and poisoning themselves, or mistakenly and incorrectly taking prescription medications. The problem might be cutting themselves, falling on a wet surface or in the tub or shower without help available, or even drowning.

As patients decline in physical and mental abilities, the house and garage should be childproofed, and slip-proofed, and the amount of supervision increased. Safeguarding or removing dangerous items, such as guns, hunting knives, chain saws, and so forth, is also necessary. Failure to realize the decline in abilities like walking can lead to dangerous situations. I am sure you have heard stories of an elderly person falling and not being able to call or get help.

Lack of Nourishment

Improper nourishment can lead to all sorts of physical and mental problems. Without careful supervision patients will neglect eating or might eat only one thing. My father-in-law would have eaten a full pound of butter in one sitting if we had let him. My own father would eat two cookies and forget that he had eaten them and in a few minutes he would be back at the cookie jar. Convincing him that he had eaten enough became a problem. The only solution was to hide the cookies.

There is a tendency to think that because they are in their last years, let them eat whatever they want. That may seem kind, but the fat in a whole pound of butter can have a major impact on the digestive system. Eating nothing but sweets or desserts can give a person a sugar high that can disrupt thought processes, prompting behavioral problems due to increased confusion. Letting someone with Alzheimer's have a glass of wine could have unwanted side effects, due to medications being taken or because of existing cognitive challenges. Seniors need good nutrition as much or more than younger people, as their bodies are not metabolizing nutrients as well. Larger portions may be needed to maintain weight, although appetites may decrease. Provide healthy snacks.

Driving

As I mentioned in the preface, I was in denial with my father. I avoided visiting him as often as I could. It was so painful to see this brilliant forest geneticist no longer able to hold long and intelligent conversations. His communication skills became that of a young child. Instead of visiting every month like I had been doing, I came every other month or every three months to visit. My mother did not receive the help from me that she needed and I missed out on being part of a team effort, as we never really created a team. Mom took on all the responsibility. One day under the stress of caring for him, my mother did not notice that my father had found the keys to the truck and had driven off. He managed to find his way home with the truck in one piece and without any scrapes or dents. Fortunately, he was safe and had not hurt anyone else.

Unfortunately, we have all read about cases in which memory patients kill or injure people while driving. Though the statistic is not high it does happen. If you are the family member whose elderly parent accidentally killed someone, you will have wished you had kept a closer eye on things. The guilt and legal responsibility can be devastating.

In the late 1970's we were gardening in the front yard of our home in Seattle. A car came down our narrow street on Queen Anne Hill. It ripped the side mirror off our truck, and sideswiped our neighbor's car, and continued to roll slowly on down the street. My husband took off running and easily caught up with the elderly man at the wheel, who was oblivious to the damage he had caused. My husband jogged alongside the car, talking to the gentleman for another half block before he convinced the driver to pull over. My husband found out where he lived and drove him home. His wife drove my husband back and surveyed the damage. She paid us and our neighbor cash and promised her husband would not get behind the wheel again. We could only hope that was the case.

Taking the keys away can become a major battle — understandably so. Losing the ability and opportunity to drive is a huge loss of independence. The best solution is to have an outside authority, like a doctor or the Department of Motor

Vehicles be the "bad guy" in telling them they can no longer drive. If a family member or friend takes on that responsibility, that person could be the target of complaints and possible aggression. Once the keys are successfully taken away, remove the vehicle. Having the car in the garage or in plain sight becomes a constant reminder of a loss of independence. Prepare yourself for many months of complaints about no longer being able to drive. Patiently listen and redirect their attention to other matters, or change the subject as quickly as possible.

Medication Dispensing and Possible Overdosing

Taking medications properly is a skill that memory patients often lose in the beginning stage of the disease. Early on in her dementia, my mother-in-law had stopped taking her medications. We thought getting a weekly pill dispenser, the kind with the days of the week labeled on it, would make it easier for her to take her medications. My husband organized all the pills and explained it to her one morning. A few days later we noticed all the pills were gone. She seemed OK, so she probably threw them out. That was when we realized we had to dispense the medications ourselves and store them in a locked cabinet.

Even if patients do not overdose, taking medications incorrectly can add to their mental confusion or cause dangerous physical side effects. Therefore, check the prescription dosage when you pick up their medications. Report any side effects to the doctor. Get rid of medications they no longer take. Keep both prescription and over-the-counter medications locked up. Dispense the medication at the same time each day to avoid complications or confusion on the part of the caregivers. A checklist taped to the inside of the locked cabinet or in a folder is a good safety measure if more than one caregiver is involved.

Neglect and/or Elder Abuse

Occasionally people do not place their loved ones in a facility because they are afraid that there might be elder abuse. The truth is that both the home and a professional care facility could be the setting for abuse. An untrained spouse or child can allow his or her temper to rage out of control when pushed to the limit by the patient. Overwhelmed, they can make detrimental decisions while trying to survive. Like a small child the elderly often can't communicate the mistreatment they are enduring. Again, this underscores the importance of objective family members educating themselves about the disease so they can properly oversee the patient's care.

Sometimes neglect or elder abuse is unintentional. Men tend to want to fix things, but memory disease is not a two-by-four that can be hammered into place. I know of a case where the husband is in denial that his wife has Alzheimer's. As a former member of the military, he believes his mission is to make her better, so she can do the dishes and housework again. Neighbors have heard this gentleman yelling at his wife in frustration, trying to motivate her to return to her household tasks. He may not be willing or able to see that he needs to assume the duties she had done in the past. His reaction here might be the result of his upbringing or cultural background. The neighbors have tried giving booklets to him, including one I wrote, *A Gradual Disappearance*, to help him face the fact that she is not going to get better. This booklet and others like it, outline how to approach memory patients by coming alongside them and entering their reality. This could be a case where the children of that couple or someone closer to the situation than the neighbors should be intervening.

Summary

As your parents age, spend more time with them. Find out what is really going on. Dad may say that everything is fine, but is he just covering up for Mom and not getting the help he needs? He may be very aware something is wrong but lack the skills or even the will to appropriately deal with the disease.

Dangers will vary from case to case. Family members will face daunting challenges as they take on the responsibility of making sure their loved one is safe and well cared for.

Chapter 3

Complications and Dangers of Denial for Family Members

The patient is not the only one at risk. Memory disease is like a spider that traps family members in its web along with the patient. It not only changes the life of the patient, but the family members' lives as well. The patient can live ten or more years with this disease. The challenges family members face will be hard enough without denial compounding problems even more. Dangers or complications can include losing the chance to make special memories, forfeiting being the best advocate for your loved one, not getting legal papers in order, family conflict, loss of financial resources for care, and stress resulting in illness or even the death of the caregivers *before* the patient passes away.

Missing Opportunities to Make Special Memories

Deep in my denial, I lost the chance to create special memories with my father, as I have been able to do with my mother. My mother is immobile and she no longer communicates more than a few words and occasionally a sentence. However, I have learned to cherish the time I do have with her. Because of our mutual love of chocolate, we enjoy a few chocolates together. Because she was a Bible Study Fellowship leader, I read Bible verses and devotionals to her. Because she was a flower show judge, I wheel her outside to look at the flowers, which she loves. Sometimes I pick a flower and place it between her fingers. I have even taken up playing the piano again, which brings a smile to her face and an occasional compliment. (Those eight years of piano lessons she paid for are finally paying off.) I try to be thankful for what we still have together, instead of concentrating on what we have lost. I can still hold her hand. If I had faced my father's dementia and created special memories with him, I would not have battled guilt over not being there for him (and Mom) during that time. I would have a chain of special memories of his last days to comfort me instead.

Forfeiting Being the Best Advocate for Your Loved One

When we were born they changed our diapers, fed us, and kept us safe. Now it is our turn to make sure our parents are properly cared for. Our spouses have loved and cared for us, and have been our partner and often our best friend. If family members do not take on this responsibility, then who is going to do it?

Recently I discussed surgery on a dementia patient with my daughter, who has a master's degree in nursing and has worked in postsurgical orthopedics for ten years. We were discussing cases of denial by family members. She reinforced the need to be objective. The hospital staff is seeing patients at their worst, in pain, strongly medicated, and in the recovery process. As the patients are going to be released, the hospital may assess that they can no longer live on their own, when in fact, they *might* be able to. An objective family member involved with a loved one's life can affirm that the patient had still been able to cook their meals, shop, and keep their house in order before the surgery.

In contrast, it is usually the hospital staff that steps in as the advocate for the memory patient, pointing out symptoms of memory disease to family members that the family has been ignoring.

By the time others can clearly see that a patient needs help, the patient is usually in the mid-stages of the disease, and family members will be playing catch-up.

The optimal situation would be if a well-orchestrated care plan were already in place due to an earlier diagnosis. Family members will have a better chance of taking needed breaks rather than wearing themselves out trying to grasp at their options for care. At the mid-stage you have most likely missed the chance to find out your loved one's end-of-life wishes. You will have to explore financial records on your own, possibly missing vital information, or face a tangled web representing an attempt at accounting. Reconstructing the current financial status could take months — time that could have been spent caring for the patient, or taking a break.

If you do not step in at the right time and become an advocate, someone else might take over that position. It could possibly be a nonfamily member or someone you do not trust. Scam artists love to prey on the elderly. Just as you would watch out for a young child, you need to start keeping an eye on the patient early on. When your loved one tells you over the phone that "everything is just fine; you don't need to stop by," you need to visit and make sure that that *is,* in fact, the case. A memory patient's idea of "just fine" may not be fine at all. If you are visiting from some distance away, talk to neighbors and local friends to get their perspective. Pay attention when they mention "new friends."

Not Getting Needed Legal Papers in Order

Another problem stemming from denial could be in not getting needed legal papers in place. Each state has different requirements and terms for the documents required. Check with your local area Agency on Aging, a lawyer, or financial planner to determine what documents you need.

These documents, sometimes called an Advanced Directive, include items such as financial power of attorney (POA), medical power of attorney, an Advanced Health Care Directive (Living Will or Physicians Orders For Life Sustaining Treatment, known as a POLST form), and written permission for adult children to see their parents' health records. Getting proper care established, dealing with finances, and authorizing needed medical procedures can be difficult without those documents in place. Social Security, the IRS, banks, wealth management companies, doctors, and even some utility companies will not allow you to manage the patient's accounts without the proper POA.

If such documents do not exist and your loved one can no longer sign or understand the documents, you would have to go to court to get legal rights to supervise their care in the form of a Conservancy. Conservatorship is expensive to initiate and maintain — not to mention the time it would take. Obtaining a conservancy also involves having your loved one publicly deemed incompetent which can be very humiliating for them. Once they are deemed incompetent they can no longer execute legal documents.

I know of a case where a stepson and his wife were trying to get care for his stepmother, who had been showing signs of Alzheimer's for some time. After being asked to help out, her biological children came from the East Coast to visit. They stayed in a hotel for a few days, took their mother out for dinner, took her shopping, and bought her a new puppy. They declared that their mother was just fine and left. The stepson was left with the same problems he had before their visit, plus a puppy, and still no legal means to get care for his stepmother.

Family Conflict

Time and time again I hear stories about families fighting over the care of a loved one: fighting over how the financial resources are spent, the type of care needed, or who is going to oversee the care. Old disagreements or grudges can resurface. Denial on the part of a family member or members can cause major family conflict. The children in denial don't help out, leaving their siblings with the burden of care. Often the ones in denial accuse their siblings of "over-reacting," thinking additional care is not needed. They might be under the illusion Mom or Dad can be retrained to make their own meals and dress themselves. Sometimes the one in denial may be the one controlling the money, which adds to the problem. I have heard of situations where one sibling has taken their parents' money for his or her own use, leaving the other siblings scrambling to find ways to finance their parents' care.

As discussed earlier, preferably, the disease should be identified at an early stage so that the patient can participate in creating a good care plan. Ideally, the care of a declining parent or spouse should be taken on as a family team effort. Sadly, "preferably" and "ideally" aren't always reality.

Loss of Financial Resources

So how are things going with your parents' finances? Oh, they have assured you many times that they have more than enough saved up for retirement. Have you been able to check out how much "more than enough" is? What if it's only ten thousand dollars for the two of them? Or you might be pleasantly surprised to find out they have a big savings account and long-term care insurance that will allow them to live in a wonderful continuing care facility for many years. That would be nice, but believing that they are taking care of everything themselves can have unfortunate results.

I was told of a case where the children were in denial that their parents needed help. When they finally faced the facts, they started looking into senior living options. They selected a facility and were in the middle of filling out paperwork when they found out their parents' stocks had all been sold at the lowest price during the last recession. Reading the newspaper stories about the recession, their father had panicked and sold everything at a major loss. They now did not have enough money for the facility they had selected.

Maybe things like this happen because your parents lived through a world war, or were raised in a culture in which the elderly hang on to their financial independence and refuse to allow family members to help. This attitude inhibits the children's ability to discover what their parents' true financial status is. Parents can dodge the issue by changing the subject or by telling their children, "It's none of your business." Even if you are being told this on a regular basis, do not give up. Respectfully and patiently assure your parents you are looking out for their best interests.

What about the property taxes? The mortgage? The utility bill? If not paid over a significant period of time, consequences could severely impact your parents' financial status.

Junk mail becomes a big issue for memory patients, as they are afraid of throwing anything away. Companies often try to make their advertising look like valid bills, so much so that it can make a person with a clear mind pause for a moment. But then, after reading a few more sentences; most of us recognize it as junk mail. A memory patient could send money to a company because they think it is a legitimate bill.

Being from another country and probably beginning to face the early fogginess of Alzheimer's, my father-in-law did not realize that as a senior citizen, he could benefit from decreased property taxes. (Not all states have this benefit.) When my husband finally took over the finances, he found out his father was paying the full property tax and immediately contacted the assessor's office. My husband applied for the discount and received it, along with reimbursement for the previous three years, which was as far back as the law would allow. We don't like to think about the previous fifteen years of taxes paid at full downtown Seattle rates.

When you are in denial, you lose the opportunity to assess how your parent's finances will support future care needs *before* there is a large demand on their assets. By not being involved, you lose the chance to make changes that might make more funds available. By putting alerts on bank accounts or limiting the amount they can withdraw, you can avoid mismanagement of funds.

Unsupervised in the early stages, patients can become the gullible victims of scam artists and telemarketers. You might ask, how can that happen?

My mother had been an astute businesswoman. She had successfully run her own dress design business before she met my father and kept it going until I was about seven or eight years old. Later, she oversaw the financial end of the family forestry ventures. When getting any work done on the house or the ranch, she normally got several bids. My parents' place, way out in the country, had a long steep driveway from the road to the house. The barns and barnyard were located on the other side of the road. The house looked out over the bay and the trees on the eighty-foot bank needed to be limbed occasionally.

Several years before she was diagnosed with Alzheimer's, my mother called me up one night quite excited. "You won't believe what happened today!" she exclaimed. "A man walked down the drive." At that point she got my attention...what kind of man would walk and not drive in? "He said that he could limb my trees on the bank for me for fifteen hundred dollars and I gave him a check for that amount and he will be back tomorrow to do the work."

I let Mom know my concerns about her not getting bids, and paying before he did the work. I hung up the phone in bewilderment. Twenty minutes later my brother called, wanting to know if I had talked to Mom. He and I did not know it yet, but we were experiencing the pre-symptomatic sign of the irrationality of Alzheimer's that often pops up several years in advance of consistent symptoms. My brother called the man and amazingly enough, he returned a few days later, with the big truck that he had left up in the barnyard on his previous visit and did the work. It became the wake-up call for my brother and me to keep a closer eye on Mom's financial decisions. Family plans regarding her care and finances had been in place for some time, but it was now time to take a more active role.

Stress Leading to Illness or Even Death

Then there is the case of the invisible patient — you, the family member. Have you discussed what you are going through with your doctor? Is your doctor aware of the stress you are under? Even if you have moved your loved one into a care facility, you are still dealing with the emotional and mental stress of overseeing their care. You still have the added pressure of being their advocate, financial planner, counselor, consoler, helper, social director, and companion. Denial will prevent you from dealing with the stress and taking the breaks you need. Watching your parent slowly decline is stressful and can lead to depression, another topic that should be discussed with your doctor. If not watched for, stress can build up and result in unusual behavior or the temporary loss of mental stability.

As her husband experienced another dramatic decline, a wife of an early-onset Alzheimer's patient was stopped by the sheriff on a country road. She had been clocked going eighty miles an hour. When stopped, she didn't even realize she was driving or where she was. Overwhelmed by the end-of-life decisions that she was having to make, she got behind the wheel without knowing what she was doing.

Recently, when facing a similar situation, I left Mom's place on my bicycle. Engrossed in my problems, I neglected to pay attention to the road. At one intersection I missed my turn from the bike lane, hit a curb almost straight on, and ended up in a bush up the side of a hill with my bike on top of me. Physically I had only a few scratches, but it was another wake-up call for me.

There is also the danger that the caregiver will die before the patient. We will discuss the invisible patient more in the next chapter.

Chapter 4

Getting Help

Another way that denial in family members plays out is in thinking professional help is not needed. Often a spouse is very aware that their husband or wife has memory disease, but they don't want anyone else to know about it. They associate shame with the disease. They lovingly try to protect their spouse from the outside world and begin to hibernate. Maybe in the beginning stages a spouse can provide the needed care, but as it snowballs, it will become overwhelming. Caring for a loved one at home is draining physically, mentally, and emotionally. However, the memory patient has an added dimension that wears the caregiver down, the dimension of unreality. The confusion seems contagious at times as you care for a loved one, day after day. It becomes a psychological game as you try to catch up to which reality he or she is in at that moment. It can be like trying to care for a two-year-old on steroids in a large body.

If your spouse or parent had heart disease and needed bypass surgery you would not attempt to do the surgery yourself. It is the same with memory disease. You will need professional help. It is hard to face the fact that someone else can give your loved one better care than you can. I have talked with spouses or children of memory patients who say, "...I know them better than anyone else; I can give them the best care." Because they are required to take continuing education classes in order to meet state licensing requirements, professional caregivers are well-trained and know the latest techniques to help your loved one.

I know from personal experience getting professional help alleviates stress. I could relax knowing that a professional caregiver was at Mom's house helping Mom dress, providing meals, giving her medications at the right time, and keeping her safe.

As a patient declines the physical care they need increases. Even if it is only a caregiver coming into the home part time, it will give you a break. You might learn new skills and ways to deal with your loved one from the caregiver. Say your mother has sundown syndrome, every afternoon about four o'clock, she becomes agitated and sometimes acts out, hitting or throwing things. An untrained person might mistakenly do things that heighten the frustration. The professional knows how to approach patients and how to distract them with an activity or music. They watch out for and minimize triggers that occur throughout the day that frustrate the patient, possibly avoiding the four o'clock meltdown altogether.

There is another reason that help is needed. Family caregivers between the ages of sixty-six and ninety-six have a 63 percent higher mortality rate than other people in the same age category — 63 percent! Caregivers often die before the loved one they are taking care of does.[8]

I know two families in which this happened and have heard about many others. In each of the two cases, it was the husband taking care of the wife with Alzheimer's or dementia. The demands on the husbands continued day and night. Both gentlemen did not let their children know what they were going through physically, mentally, and emotionally. Even though one husband had no previous history of heart disease, he got so worn out he had a heart attack. The other gentleman had become so worn out and sleep deprived that he contracted a serious infection. After several falls, he developed other complications that his depleted body could not fight. Both gentlemen passed away about the same time.

In both cases, the children had to step in and care for Mom immediately. With no plan in place, after providing approximately a week of care, the siblings were so worn out they could not function. In one of the cases, four healthy adults in their sixties could not keep up the pace their ninety-year-old father had been trying to keep. Both families had to quickly find a facility for their mothers, and oversee the care for their fathers as they were dying. These stressful situations could have been avoided if the fathers had reached out for help earlier.

The greatest generation — the members of the WWII era are not accustomed to asking for help. The men especially seem to be used to keeping bad situations private, solving their own problems, and helping others but not asking for help themselves. These and other factors are why we can end up with parents who will not let us into their world as they start to decline. It is a problem I hear about all the time. Of the families mentioned above, in one case, the children had tried to reach out to their father to help. He let them bring in a weekly meal and do a little housecleaning, but he still kept up a good front, not allowing them to guess how much time and attention his wife demanded. Breaking down those barriers can be hard because at the same time, we want to respect our parents' privacy and promote any independence that they might still have. Sometimes a good social worker or a representative from the Council on Aging can help break down those barriers.

Moving my mother into a memory care facility was like a vacation for me. It freed me from the daily responsibilities and I could spend time with Mom again. Before that, my weekly visit to her place outside of Olympia, Washington was consumed with checking on things in the house; taking her to town for her hair appointment; picking up meds, supplies, and groceries; going over the mail; and paying the bills. The schedule did not allow much time to talk or enjoy each other's company. Whether I was back at my home in California, living on our boat in Seattle, or on the plane between homes, I would make up lists and schedules for the caregivers and go over paperwork for the house or for her medical needs. It was non-stop. Once Mom moved into a facility, many bills became one monthly bill to pay. I could use the time I had spent making up schedules for the caregivers to put a puzzle together with her or wheel her around the garden. She stopped calling me "Mother" and began introducing me as her daughter again.

It is important to reach out and get professional help and good advice, which will give you peace of mind. Then you will make better choices for your loved one.

Chapter 5

Level of Care

So we accept the fact our loved one has memory disease. We have secured proper care for him or her. There is still another area in which we can slip into denial. That comes when the level of care is changing or has changed. The progression of memory disease is a sporadic decline. Sometimes it is a slow one and other times a fast one. Patients can have months of getting slightly better. It's like a roller coaster coming into the last part of the ride: up and down, but always descending.

Each step down can be hard to accept. We can easily stick our head in the sand again. I had trouble accepting my mother's move into a shared room. We started looking into moving Mom into a shared room for financial reasons and were surprised by the encouragement of the staff. They felt she would do better with a roommate. The day we moved her out of her single room into the double I could hardly keep from crying as we worked. As the facilities crew left, I looked around her new room: all the furniture was in place, the bed was looking good with new pillows, and a tapestry Mom wove many years before was hanging above her bed. I was ready to go upstairs and get Mom from the hair salon and bring her to her new room when the director of the memory care unit walked in. He commented about how nice it looked and the next thing I knew I was sobbing in his arms. I regained my composure and on the way to the elevator, I was kicking myself. What was my problem? This was ridiculous. Why carry on like that? As I wheeled Mom to her new room I realized I didn't want to face the fact that her personal space was shrinking, that she was declining.

Then over the next week, Mom blossomed. I would ask her how she liked her roommate, whose bed was about six feet from hers. She would look at me, smile and say, "Oh, I don't have a roommate." The caregivers would tell me they would often hear her and her roommate chatting for a few minutes after they got into bed for the night. They liked having the company.

A marketing director told me she was working late in the assisted living facility where she was employed at the time. The facility did not offer memory care, and many of the residents were showing signs of dementia. Some had declined to the point they needed 24/7 supervision. The day staff had left, and there was only the skeleton crew for the night shift. There was a lady meandering through the halls, dressed to go out shopping, purse and all. The marketing director found a nighttime caregiver to help the lady back to her room. Several other evenings she found confused residents wandering into the kitchen or near the front door. When she looked into these cases, she found family members who were resisting the staff's suggestions that their loved one be moved to a memory care facility.

Not accepting that your loved one has declined to another level of care can be dangerous. Ignoring the fact that Dad needs a walker can lead to a fall, resulting in broken bones, displaced joints, hospitalization, and the use of pain medication. Being on certain medication can cause significant mental and physical decline for the elderly. Sometimes it may be temporary or it may be permanent.

Not facing the fact that Dad needs more supervision has other ramifications. He may begin falling, have more agitation episodes, attempt to run away, or develop depression.

By way of illustration, I met a family as they were moving their mother, Sue, (as I will call her) into assisted living. Sue hibernated in her room, refusing to eat. Two of her daughters took turns spending the night with her. Other family members tried to help their mother adjust to the move. Sue kept sliding deeper into depression, refusing to go to activities or to eat in the dining room. The staff kept suggesting that the family take their mother to visit the memory care wing, but they balked at that idea. Finally, after almost a month, they agreed. At first Sue would just visit the memory care wing for lunch or a few activities. Then she began participating and interacting with the other residents. She began eating again. She felt at home in memory care. Assisted living was overwhelming for her.

As mentioned in an earlier chapter, not facing the fact that a loved one is declining can be financially detrimental. Not providing additional supervision when needed can have repercussions. Many Alzheimer's patients become paranoid. Memories and stories of the Great Depression are fresh in their minds as they are often living in their childhood. Trusting a bank or loved ones becomes difficult for them. This can result in them closing bank accounts and hiding the money. Then the guessing game becomes one of where did they hide it, or worse, what did they spend it on? If it is an account with automatic deposits or withdrawals, there are additional problems. Failure to supervise financial affairs allows problems to mushroom even further if not caught quickly. Late fees, loss of utilities, and even the loss of their home could occur.

Chapter 6

Struggling to Understand

When our loved one becomes more and more of a stranger to us, we naturally want to understand where their mind is. What are they thinking? Do they recognize who we are? Sometimes they let us in for a while with their words or actions and if we patiently observe, we can guess what it is they want. Extreme patience is required as it might take them a while to communicate via their eyes, grunts and groans, hand gestures, and maybe confused verbiage.

My father used to tell my mother, "You have no idea what I am going through." The despair and confusion in his eyes haunted her for a long time. Now I sometimes see the same despair and confusion in my mother's eyes as she struggles to communicate even one word to me. Up until recently, she smiled when she saw me and would often laugh. Over the last six months, her bubbly personality has subsided, and often her tired eyes stare blankly into space. I hope her mind has taken her somewhere pleasant.

Earlier we mentioned aggressive or violent behavior. What triggers acting out? "If you don't understand what's happening because your brain is not functioning, it can be scary," says Beth Kallmyer, senior director of constituent services at the Alzheimer's Association. "It's normal human behavior. You might act out, become agitated, or violent if you don't know what's going on." [9]

If you stay objective, you might be able to figure out what is triggering this aggression. What is your loved one afraid of or confused by? When she still lived in her home, my mother used to be terrified and talk about gangs of men on the road. If we said we couldn't see them, she would become angry. Trees had grown over the years and blocked the view of the road. I learned to agree that I could see them and then say something like, "Oh, look, Mom, they have turned around and they are leaving." The problem was now resolved and she could relax.

Nancy Nelson, the poet I mentioned earlier, has given me permission to share one of her poems. She has given us a gift in sharing a personal insight into the thoughts of an Alzheimer's patient. Her book, *Blue. River. Apple.* is now available on Amazon. It is a vivid, sometimes blunt description of what she has been facing. She is attempting to face Alzheimer's head on.

Blue. River. Apple.

Today's Journey:
Develop courage,
Splash on a smile,
Be who I want to be.
Not afraid of who I am becoming.

To awake at night, fearful of forgetting
Important and precious things like...
People. Dates. Times. Appointments.
I am not in control. Please help me, God.

Thoughts jumble, words disappear.
Times mix up, promises go astray.
When I hear, "Where are you?" "Are you coming?"
Eyes water, stomach churns, humbled in disbelief.
I know I have done it again!

Do I stay home, cancel, quit?
Or fight for right of passage through the fog?
Silently, I say, I am not what I appear.
I am sorry for what you see.

Breathe in courage,
Splash on a smile,
Struggle to remember ...
I must find pieces of myself and revel in who I know I am.
Chin up, treading lightly in new uncharted waters.

At times, I catch sideways glances, back and forth.
Perhaps, even, your voice impatient. I understand.
But, wait, we stand together, separate.
Can you hear me? I have so much to tell you.

I try to mask the imperfections.
A dab of foundation, a blush of pink.
Dressed in clothes, jewelry, and resolve
Daily, though, I have to make sense of where I am.

On the sliding scale of … Blue. River. Apple.

I want to be Positive.
I am Productive.
I am Loving and Beloved.
I am Grateful, Creative, Alive.
Therefore …
I am blessed with a voice to tell my inner story.

Blue. River. Apple.

Never assume your loved one cannot understand. At times my
mother will say a few words that prove she is very aware of the
current conversation. When she could speak fluently, it was
apparent that her reality was constantly changing between the
present, the past, or some make-believe situation. She would
say something so apropos, and then ask if I saw my father (who
passed away over twenty-five years ago) in the hall, explaining
that he had just brought her some beautiful flowers.

So as our loved ones decline to the point they cannot communicate, we must not assume they do not understand. We
have to be careful not to speak about them as if they are not

there. Always communicate when with them as if they are a vital part of the conversation.

An exception would be conversations about end-of-life or medical conditions with a doctor, a professional, or other family members. These conversations should take place in another room, not in front of patients as if they do not exist.

Chapter 7

Survival

When we are dealing with a disease that robs us of our loved ones, causes confusion, a lack of communication, and unhappiness...how can we survive?

Caregiver Gary Joseph LeBlanc in his September 27, 2011, post for the Fisher Center for Alzheimer's website suggests:

> If possible, a family meeting should be held right after the initial diagnosis is obtained. The sooner everyone realizes that their loved ones will no longer be able to care for themselves in the near future, the less denial will be brought forward. Even if this gathering becomes a one-time event (which it shouldn't), it's vital that family members become aware of how extreme the situation truly is. Hopefully they will recognize how unfair it is to drop everything into only one person's lap. [10]

Getting the family to work together is the ideal situation. It will keep people from burning-out while overseeing the care of the memory patient. Unfortunately too often it all comes back to one person. Try to find ways to incorporate everyone as a team, and put a flexible plan in place. Trusted family members who live far away can oversee the finances online, pay bills, etcetera. They can also do needed research online for care options, doctors, caregivers, and senior living facilities. Think of each family member's strengths to find areas where that person can help. It's not just your loved one's personal care and safety you have to worry about; there are income and property taxes, taking care of or preparing to sell the home, medical forms, social security forms, keeping up with changes in Medicare, friends of your loved one to correspond with, and their organizations or religious groups to contact.

With smartphones, tablets, and social media, there are all sorts of ways friends and family members who live far away can participate in making this journey a more pleasant one. Facetime, Skype, or showing photos on a larger screen like a tablet might help break up the patient's day and help keep their mind in a positive place. For my mother, seeing photos on a smartphone has been confusing. However, she does relate to the larger photos on my tablet. Playing her favorite songs on a playlist as I feed her helps lighten the mood. On her good days, I also call family and friends on speaker mode so that she can hear their voices. Occasionally, she will join in on the conversation.

Caring for my mother has been easier than it was caring for my in-laws. This is not only because we know a lot more about what we are doing and we have a bigger budget, but also because we know what she wants. My mother gave us the gift of getting all her financial and medical papers in place and also talking about how she wanted to be cared for. She planned her burial and even wrote down facts for her obituary. She let us know that she did not want us taking on her physical care ourselves. She watched my husband and me providing the physical care for my in-laws, and when we were alone, she would say, "I never want to be like that, but if I am, I don't want you to care for me. I want you to put me someplace and forget about me; go on with your own lives."

I obeyed part of her wishes. When she declined to the point she could not stay in her home, I researched and found wonderful care for her near my house so that I can visit almost every day, feed her meals and spend time with her. We know that she does not want to be kept alive "through extraordinary measures" and she proved it by signing three different end-of-life directives. There are not any arguments between my brother and me about her care or end-of-life wishes. This is the advantage of end-of-life discussions with your loved ones while they are still coherent.

Another way to survive is humor. It always helps to make light of a bad situation. Memory patients still love a good joke. Mom and I love to watch HGTV together as she always loved redecorating her home. Yet, it's the commercials that provide the most humor. I make comments about the little kids or joke about situations, and she smiles. There is a commercial about Alaska that says, "Where your neighbors are bald and hibernate half the year." I mentioned that the bald eagle looked like a certain family member, and she laughed and laughed. Humor is a great stress reliever for all parties concerned.

Creating fun memories is a survival tool. Celebrate the big occasions like birthdays, grandkids' graduations, or other happy times. If your love one can't attend they can still talk on the phone and see videos or photos of the occasion. Take them out to the park, out to eat, or for a walk if possible. They may not remember, but you will, and it will lift your spirits.

Taking a break is also an important tool in making this journey a gratifying or pleasant one. Get away from the situation, do something you enjoy, join a support group. Taking a break is a good way to stay more objective. Without respites, family caregivers can become like a frog in a pot on the stove, not realizing that the water, which started out nice and cool, is now close to boiling. Family caregivers commonly experience depression, fatigue, and illness. When you are rested, you will be able to make better decisions concerning your loved one's care. By taking care of yourself, you are taking care of those you love.

Don't take things personally. Assign blame to the disease for aggressive, rude, or unpleasant behavior. Don't assume it is any dislike for you. When a loved one says something mean or tries to hit or bite you, remember it is not really that person's true nature; it is the disease.

My husband got a chuckle out of his father's perception of life one morning. My father-in-law had been explaining to my husband all about his farm in Norway that his son ran and how successful this son was. My husband had to keep from laughing, as he is an only child and his uncle owned the family farm in Norway, not my father-in-law. Finding this story amusing, my husband asked his father more about his son. After listening to more of this fantasy, he asked, "So who am I?"

My father-in-law quickly answered, "Oh, you're the hired help."

Likewise, my mother also had to learn to not take offense at my father's insistence that he needed a new, *younger* wife. I knew this was not my father talking, as he would tell people over the forty years of their marriage, that if he had met Mom in first grade he would have found a way to marry her by second grade. His love for her was unquestionable.

Support groups are lifesavers. Having someone else to talk to who is going through the same thing alleviates some of the loneliness that comes with caregiving. Learning that fear, sadness, and anger are normal emotions when traveling this path helps. Being able to share with others something your loved one did that you think is bizarre and having them say, "Yes, my mother did that, too," gives relief as you realize oddity is normal with memory disease. Sharing funny stories about what your loved one said or did with someone who understands that you are not making fun of your loved one, but you have to laugh about it or you will break down and cry, brings comfort. And sometimes, finding another shoulder to cry on, either figuratively or literally, helps dispel some of the stress.

I cannot emphasize enough how important it is to get professional help. It is necessary to survive because, as the disease progresses, the amount of help necessary will increase. The National Alzheimer's Association and the Chronic Care Consortium collaborated to provide a list called *The Six Stages of Caregiving for Alzheimer's Patients*. The stages they outline are Pre-diagnostic, Diagnostic, Role Change, Chronic Caregiving, Transition to Alternative Care, and End of Life. This article carefully outlines the decline of the patient and the added caregiving the patient will need. While it is a good outline and follows the common path most Alzheimer's patients take, each case varies as the disease attacks each patient's brain differently. The Alzheimer's Association website alz.org also has extensive description of the three stages of Alzheimer's, informing caregivers on what to expect. [11]

Alzheimer's is a cruel disease at the end of life. Depending on which part of the brain it attacks, some patients cannot stop yelling or trying to hit those around them. Others, like my father-in-law, lose the use of motor skills and forget how to walk. Those who don't die of other health problems may eventually starve to death or die of complications of pneumonia. My husband is still haunted by the memory of his father taking a bite of food and then starting to cry, as he could no longer remember how to chew or swallow.

If you are a person of faith, I would encourage you to reach out to your church, temple, or another group for support and strength. My husband and I know that much of our support came from the prayers of fellow Christians.

Chapter 8

How to Overcome or Help Others Overcome Denial

How can you help yourself, a family member or a friend in denial? First you should determine if it is just a matter of someone needing a little more time to adjust to the fact that Mom or Dad or their spouse has memory disease. This can be shocking news as it is so personal. Your sibling could be thinking, "If Mom has dementia, I could be next!" Denial can be a good stopgap measure if it is softening the initial shock; it is staying in denial that is harmful.

Keeping a journal can be a positive way to overcome denial. Writing down your fears or aversions can help you face them and help you identify any irrational beliefs or responses you might have.

Seeking out a friend, a loved one, or a professional to talk to about your denial can help you overcome it. Again, support groups can help, as other people taking the same journey will understand what you are going through. Allow yourself to share your fears and emotions.

When family members or friends appear to be stuck in denial, try to determine the root cause of the denial. This disease can bring out a whole spectrum of emotions in family members. Is it fear, anger, or pain? Are they afraid of the disease or afraid it might happen to them? Is there a history of a falling out with the family member with memory disease, and they don't want to face the responsibility? Is it too painful to face a loved one who has such an illness, and by denying it, they are avoiding pain?

After reviewing several lists by specialists, including one by Carol Larkin, a geriatric care manager on how to help someone overcome denial, I decided to write my own list based on my experiences with caregiving. Here are some ideas to help you talk to others about denial:

1) Attitude is everything; show kindness, be calm, and try to understand their frame of reference. Ask them to share with you how they see the problem. Make them feel secure enough to share their feelings by providing a sympathetic ear and understanding spirit.

2) Try to figure out what is triggering their denial. Let them know that fear, anger, pain, helplessness, or whatever emotion they are experiencing is normal, but allowing that emotion to take over does not help them or their loved one. Help them honestly examine the emotion that is causing the denial.

3) Let them know that you will be there for them. Emphasize the need for teamwork and how much they are needed on the team. Talk about potential negative consequences if a plan for care is not put into place.

4) Explore any irrational beliefs, like wondering if they might catch the disease. Help them realize the fallacy of these beliefs.

5) Talk about the goal of providing the best care for the loved one. Even though it might be inconvenient or they might be justifiably angry with the loved one, it is the right thing to do.

6) Explain that doing nothing will only allow the problem to blossom into a much larger one.

7) Don't argue with them. If they are not open to discussion, change the subject and bring it up at a later time.

Hearing the words "dementia" or "Alzheimer's" can overwhelm some people, especially if they are already carrying a heavy load in providing for someone else. Like drinking too much or taking drugs, denial does not solve any problems. Denial only alleviates the pain for a time, if at all.

I am constantly telling others to research the disease. Go to alz.org, or the Mayo Clinic website (http://www.mayoclinic.org) Find other reputable sites. This will not only arm you with information to make your journey easier, but also becomes a tool in overcoming denial. With more information you might find you have blown some things way out of proportion. You will learn how to deal with aspects of the disease that might scare or revolt you. You will learn where to turn to for help. Do the research, and let the denial slip away.

Conclusion

I want to encourage you to stay objective, get the facts, and take time for yourself. Be like the ostrich; compassionate, caring, observant, and resourceful.

Show compassion for the people affected by memory disease, for other family members walking the same path, for the caregivers who are dealing with difficult patients, and for those in denial. Find ways you can lend a hand in making someone's journey easier. A giving, loving spirit will always make your own burden lighter.

Carefully assess the situation your loved one is in. How can it be improved? What are potential dangers? How can you prepare for future needs? Put all the knowledge you have gained through research toward solutions. For example, if you notice your loved one's motor skills are diminishing, find out if Medicare will cover a walker or wheelchair, what your responsibilities will be in obtaining the equipment, if renting equipment is the best solution, and so forth.

Maintaining objectivity is an essential key to making the journey easier.

Take breaks and make sure you are looking after your own health: eat a Mediterranean diet, exercise, keep your weight down, and use your brain.

Scientists are conducting studies concerning genetic predisposition for Alzheimer's. If this is a concern, go to alz.org and click the "Life with Alz" tab to find a wealth of information on how to ease the effects of Alzheimer's.

Often people ask me what has been my key to surviving this journey four times. The answer is by keeping my eyes on my Lord and Savior, Jesus Christ. Through prayer and God's Word I have found peace and the strength to continue. Dr. Sameh Elsanadi, a Geriatric Psychologist in Orange County, California, has told me that he has observed that families of faith do much better dealing with this disease.

During my four journeys, I have learned to be more patient, to slow down, and to enjoy the moment.

Remember that like anything in life, this journey is all about your attitude. I will close with this quote by author Melody Beattie: "Gratitude unlocks the fullness of life. It turns what we have into enough, and more it turns denial into acceptance, chaos to order, confusion to clarity. It can turn a meal into a feast, a house into a home, a stranger into a friend." [12]

Find even the smallest things to be grateful for, and the journey will become a meaningful one with moments of joy.

Definitions

M erriam – *Webster's* definition of Alzheimer's:
A degenerative brain disease of unknown cause that is the most common form of dementia, that usually starts in late middle age or in old age, that results in progressive memory loss, impaired thinking, disorientation, and changes in personality and mood, and that is marked histologically by the degeneration of brain neurons especially in the cerebral cortex and by the presence of neurofibrillary tangles and plaques containing beta-amyloid — called also *Alzheimer's*. [13]

Alzheimer's Association's definition of Alzheimer's:

Alzheimer's disease is a progressive brain disorder that damages and eventually destroys brain cells, leading to loss of memory, thinking and other brain functions. Alzheimer's is not a part of normal aging, but results from a complex pattern of abnormal changes. It usually develops slowly and gradually gets worse as more brain cells wither and die. Ultimately, Alzheimer's is fatal, and currently, there is no cure.

Alzheimer's disease is the most common type of *dementia,* a general term used to describe various diseases and conditions that damage brain cells. Alzheimer's disease accounts for 50 to 80 percent of dementia cases. Other types include vascular dementia, mixed dementia, dementia with Lewy bodies and frontotemporal dementia.[14]

Mayo Clinic definition of dementia:

Dementia isn't a specific disease. Instead, dementia describes a group of symptoms affecting intellectual and social abilities severely enough to interfere with daily functioning. Many causes of dementia symptoms exist. Alzheimer's disease is the most common cause of a progressive dementia.

Memory loss generally occurs in dementia, but memory loss alone doesn't mean you have dementia. Dementia indicates problems with at least two brain functions, such as memory loss and impaired judgment or language. Dementia can make you confused and unable to remember people and names. You also may experience changes in personality and social behavior. However, some causes of dementia are treatable and even reversible.[15]

Merriam-Webster's definition of dementia:

A usually progressive condition (as Alzheimer's disease) marked by deteriorated cognitive functioning often with emotional apathy.[16]

Suggested Resources

A Place for Mom: http://www.aplaceformom.com
Caregivers.com: http://caregiver.com/channels/alz/
Catholic Community Services: Google search for your local chapter
Hospice Net: www.hospicenet.org/html/find.html
National Council for the Aging: www.ncoa.org/
The Alzheimer's Association: http://www.alz.org
The Mayo Clinic: http://www.mayoclinic.org

Suggested Reading

A Gradual Disappearance by Elizabeth Lonseth. An introductory support booklet for family members dealing with a loved one with Alzheimer's or dementia.

Blue. River. Apple. - an exploration of Alzheimer's through poetry by Nancy Nelson, an Alzheimer's patient. It gives insight from her viewpoint of this journey.

Letters from Madelyn, Chronicles of a Caregiver by Elaine K. Sanchez. A compilation of letters written to Elaine from her mother, Madelyn. It details the day-to-day challenges of being a caregiver.

Still Alice by Lisa Genova. Written from the perspective of the patient dealing with early-onset dementia.

The Circle by Sally Hughes Smith. A daughter's journal account of the emotions dealt with when she moved her mother into a memory care facility from her childhood home.

The Emotional Survival Guide for Caregivers: Looking After Yourself and Your Family While Helping an Aging Parent by Barry J. Jacobs PsyD (Guilford, 2006). A compassionate book by an expert to help caregiving families avoid burnout.

Endnotes

1 Alzheimer's Association, 10 Early Signs and Symptoms of Alzheimer's, 2015. Retrieved from http://www.alz.org/alzheimers_disease_10_signs_of_alzheimers.asp

2 Alzheimer's Association, 2015 Alzheimer's Disease Facts & Figures. Retrieved from http://www.alz.org/facts/overview.asp

3 *New Study Ranks Alzheimer's as Third Leading Cause of Death* by Tara Bahrampour, The Washington Post, March 15, 2014. Retrieved from http://www.washington-post.com/local/new-study-ranks-alzheimers-as-third-leading-cause-of-death-after-heart-disease-and-cancer/2014/03/05/8097a452-a48a-11e3-8466-d34c451760b9_story.html

4 Washington tops U.S. in 12-year Alzheimer's Death Rates by Matt Rosenberg, Social Capital Review, March 28th, 2013. Retrieved from http://socialcapitalreview.org/?s=Washington+top+US+in+12-year+Alzheimer%27s+death+rates and World Life Expectancy website, USA Alzheimer's Life Expectancy. Retrieved from http://www.worldlifeexpectancy.com/usa-cause-of-death-by-age-and-gender

5 *Wikipedia*, s.v. "Sundowning, dementia)," last modified March 1, 2015, http://en.wikipedia.org/wiki/Sundowning

6 *Aggression and Violence in patients with dementia*, by Dr. Jaya Joy and Dr. Joe John Vattakatucher, GM (Geriatric Medicine) April 2013 Journal. Retrieved from https://www.gmjournal.co.uk/aggression_and_violence_in_patients_with_dementia_78559.aspx

7 10 Alternative Ways to Say No to Someone with Dementia, by Paula Spenser Scott, Caring.com contributing editor. Retrieved from https://www.caring.com/articles/10-alternative-ways-to-say-no-to-someone-with-dementia

8 Family Caregiver Alliance Website, Caregiver Health, Caregivers pay the ultimate price for providing care — increased mortality. Retrieved from https://caregiver.org/caregiver-health

9 *When Alzheimer's Turns Violent* by Madison Park, CNN, March 30, 2011. Retrieved from http://edition.cnn.com/2011/HEALTH/03/30/alzheimers.violence.caregiving/

10 *Battling the Denial of Alzheimer's* by Gary Joseph LeBlanc, Post for the Fisher Center for Alzheimer's. September 27,2011. Retrieved from https://www.alzinfo.org/treatment-care/blogs/2011/09/battling-denial-alzheimers/

11 Stages of Alzheimer's, Alzheimer's Association, Retrieved from http://alz.org/alzheimers_disease_stages_of_alzheimers.asp

12 Quote by Author Melody Beattie, Brainy Quotes. Retrieved from www.brainyquote.com/quotes/authors/m/melody_beattie.html

13 "Alzheimer's" (2012). In Merriam-Webster Dictionary. Retrieved from www.merriam-webster.co./dictionary/Alzheimer's

14 "Alzheimer's" (2012). At Alzheimer's Association website. Retrieved from www.alz.org/research/science/alzheimers

15 "Dementia" (1998-2012). At Mayo Clinic website. Retrieved from www.mayoclinic.com/health/dementia

16 "Dementia" (2012). In Merriam-Webster Dictionary. Retrieved from www.merrian-webster.com/dictionary/dementia

Other Books by Elizabeth Lonseth

Non Fiction
A Gradual Disappearance

Christian Fiction
Leave It With Him
Cares Of This World

50339349R10043

Made in the USA
San Bernardino, CA
20 June 2017